FAQ

TEEN LIFE™

FREQUENTLY ASKED QUESTIONS ABOUT

Avian Flu

Jeanne
Nagle

ROSEN
PUBLISHING®
New York

Published in 2009 by The Rosen Publishing Group, Inc.
29 East 21st Street, New York, NY 10010

Library of Congress Cataloging-in-Publication Data

Nagle, Jeanne.
Frequently asked questions about avian flu / Jeanne Nagle.
      p. cm.—(FAQ: teen life)
ISBN-13: 978-1-4042-1810-9 (library binding)
1. Avian influenza. I. Title.
RA644.I6N34 2007
636.5'0896203—dc22

                                                    2008010301

Manufactured in the United States of America

Contents

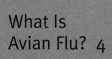

WHAT IS AVIAN FLU?

These days, evening news reports, Internet chatter, newspaper headlines, and magazine covers are abuzz about avian, or bird, flu. But what exactly is bird flu?

The term "avian flu" generally refers to an infection by the type A (H5N1) influenza virus. The "H" and the "N" in the official name H5N1 are protein markers that explain to scientists how the virus reproduces and infects other cells.

Wild birds are often infected by the influenza A (H5N1) virus. Though it resides in their intestines, they rarely get sick from it. However, they can pass the virus to domesticated birds such as chickens, turkeys, and ducks. These birds are much more vulnerable to the virus and often get sick and die when infected.

More severe strains of the virus can result in a nearly 100 percent mortality (death) rate in domesticated poultry.

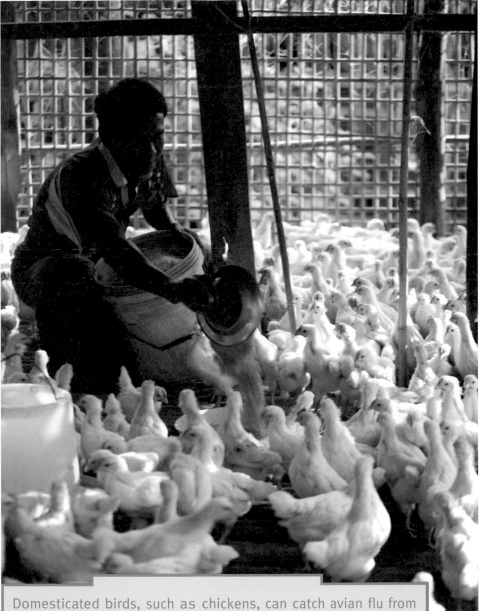

Domesticated birds, such as chickens, can catch avian flu from wild birds. The disease spreads quickly among chickens and can be passed from them to humans, especially to those who handle the birds.

Research has shown that H5N1 has been growing more powerful, becoming more dangerous to wild waterfowl and even some mammals.

Bird Flu in Humans

It is not easy for humans to become infected with the virus. Most of those who have become ill came into contact with bird feces (solid waste), urine, saliva, or other secretions. Symptoms are similar to ordinary flu symptoms—cough, fever, aches, breathing difficulty, sore throat, pneumonia—but they develop faster and are more severe. Studies have shown that avian flu can be transported from one place to another via clothing, shoes, or even tractor wheels. Anyone who kills, de-feathers, butchers, or prepares an infected bird is at high risk. Open-air markets where people sell chickens are considered hotbeds of infection.

Despite all this, it is extremely rare for the virus to be passed from person to person. Furthermore, there has never been a documented case of person-to-person-to-person transmission, meaning the virus does not seem to continue on to a third person after a second person is infected.

The number of human cases of avian flu has increased over the last several years, since the first documented case in 1997. Given the number of birds that have the virus, however, the number of humans infected remains quite low. Because of these factors, the possibility of widespread infection is greatly reduced.

Threat of a Pandemic

There are fears that avian flu could spread across the globe, infecting and killing thousands or even millions of humans in a deadly pandemic. A pandemic is a global outbreak of a disease, often spreading easily from person to person. However, the truth is considerably less alarming. At this point, you have little chance of contracting avian flu, especially if you do not handle birds or come into contact with uncooked poultry very often.

Still, scientists fear the virus may mutate in such a way that person-to-person transmission will become easier, leading to the possibility of an epidemic or pandemic. Preparations are being made for this worst-case scenario. Epidemiologists (who study the causes of diseases and the way they spread) and other researchers are working overtime to test effective medications and develop a vaccine that will prevent infection in the first place.

This is by no means the first deadly global flu scare in history and it won't be the last. Keep in mind that very few of these scares have emerged as the deadly scourge they were initially feared to be.

WHAT ARE VIRUSES AND PANDEMICS?

To truly understand the extent and gravity of a potential pandemic like avian flu, you first must have a basic understanding of biology and the fundamentals of how a virus works.

What Is a Virus?

A virus is made up of three elements: nucleic acid (DNA or RNA) that contains the virus's genetic instructions; a membrane that surrounds the nucleic acid; and a protein capsid that encloses the nucleic acid-membrane composite. Viruses are very tiny, about one-millionth of an inch long, but they can cause major damage to organisms, including humans.

Viruses typically invade living things such as animals or humans through the host's nose, mouth, or broken skin. Once inside, they target and bind themselves to cells, eventually getting inside the cells and harvesting cellular

Below are two avian influenza viruses, seen at 108,000x magnification.

machinery to make more or new viruses or virus particles. These particles gather together to form new viruses, which then break free from the host cell, often destroying it in the process. They then move on to infect other healthy cells and repeat the process until the host is full of disease.

Viruses can also mutate. They go in, grab genes of other viruses already present in the host, and alter their own genetic code in the process. Mutation gives them new tools with which to infect a host, as well as extra strength to resist and survive standard treatments because they keep changing and drugs aren't always effective against them any longer. Mutations also help viruses "leap" from animal to human populations.

The way a virus spreads depends on what type it is. The most common methods are through:

- Carrier organisms (mosquitoes, birds, etc.)
- The air/aerosol
- Direct transfer of body fluids from one person to another (saliva, sweat, nasal secretions, blood, etc.)
- Surfaces on which these body fluids have been

Viruses are not the same as bacteria. Viruses are single cells and cannot reproduce on their own. They have to invade the cells of a host in order to replicate. Viruses cause illnesses such as AIDS, hepatitis, and Ebola. All types of influenza are viruses. Bacteria, on the other hand, are the smallest living organisms.

Type A Flu Viruses

Influenza viruses are divided into three types, depending on their structure. They are called A, B, and C. While B and C affect humans only, A can infect both animals and people. C is considered rather mild, while type A can be the lethal kind. Type B can also be quite serious.

Type A viruses are further identified by two subtypes of cell surface proteins: hemagglutinin (HA) and neuraminidase (NA). There are fifteen strains of hemagglutinin and nine strains of neuraminidase. These strains are constantly evolving through two different processes. Antigenic drift involves small, permanent, ongoing changes in the genetic material of a virus strain, while antigenic shift involves sudden, major changes.

Avian flu is a type A virus and is extremely dangerous. It can mutate directly or indirectly into a human flu.

How Pandemics Occur

Human pandemics usually start as viruses in the animal world. From there, the virus mutates to where it becomes a new subtype of an existing virus, one that can infect the human population.

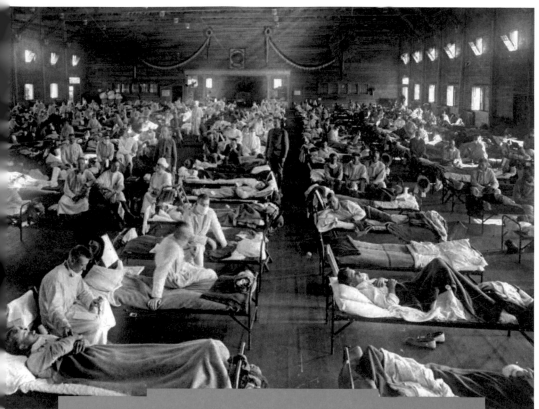

Above, Spanish influenza patients rest at an emergency hospital in Kansas in 1918. The 1918 Spanish influenza pandemic killed approximately twenty million people worldwide.

The new virus easily infects people, making them seriously ill. It is very contagious. Pandemics often come in waves, spaced weeks to months apart.

Pandemics consist of six distinct phases. In phase one, a new virus subtype is present in animals, but the risk of human infection is low. Phase two is when an animal virus begins to pose a risk to humans of contracting the disease. A new subtype virus may infect humans in phase three, but there is little or no chance of human-to-human spread. When phase four begins, spread of the virus is localized, meaning it is relatively contained and is not well-adapted to humans. It becomes more adapted by phase five, even though it's not fully able to be transmitted from one person to another. Phase six is a full-on pandemic, where a virus spreads easily throughout the general population from human to human.

Avian flu is currently considered to be in phase three.

three

WHAT ARE SOME OF HISTORY'S PANDEMICS?

Pandemics are nothing new. Reports of them date as far back as 430 BCE. Influenza pandemics, however, were not first recorded until 1889.

Past influenza pandemics led to high death tolls. It is the memory of these past killers that has many people fearful now. However, avian flu's progress is being carefully monitored, and our twenty-first-century world is in a much better position to stave off a catastrophe. By taking the time to study history's pandemics carefully, experts can learn vital lessons about how to prepare for the next one.

The Spanish Flu of 1918

During World War I, Fort Riley, Kansas, was home to twenty-six thousand soldiers. In the spring of 1918, hundreds of soldiers showed up at the fort's infirmary, complaining of sore throat, fever, and deep cough. Soon their lungs shut down completely. Soldiers died before doctors even determined what was wrong with them.

The problem not only persisted, it spread. Soon, other military camps around the world were being hit by this illness. When Spain's King Alphonse III fell victim, updates on his condition were broadcast around the world. Since Spain was the first nation to announce officially the presence of this new disease, it quickly became known as the Spanish Lady, or the Spanish flu.

By early summer, the Spanish flu had traveled far beyond the United States and western Europe to Russia, North Africa, India, China, Japan, and New Zealand. It had killed tens of thousands of people. Then, just as mysteriously as the flu appeared, it disappeared at summer's end. People believed the worst was over.

Sadly, they were wrong. A second wave was on its way. In the fall, the Spanish flu returned with a vengeance. The U.S. Department of Health had no choice but to issue a public warning that an epidemic was underway.

The Spanish flu was fast moving and deadly. Tens of thousands of people died in every major city around the world. The only continent not affected was Antarctica. Estimates of the number of fatalities worldwide ranged widely, between twenty million and one hundred million.

Researchers have studied the preserved remains of some of the victims of the 1918 flu pandemic to discover just why this particular virus killed so many so fast. Their conclusion is that the Spanish flu was a type of virus that humans had never encountered before, so they had no immunity to it. They also

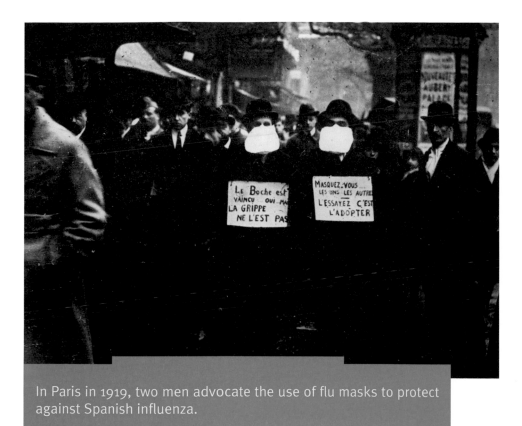

In Paris in 1919, two men advocate the use of flu masks to protect against Spanish influenza.

discovered that it was a type A virus—the most fatal—that first occurred in birds and mutated in such a way that it could leap to humans and infect them.

The Asian Flu and the Hong Kong Flu

In the late 1950s, the Asian flu was sweeping the world. First identified in northern China early in 1957, it reached the United States during the summer of that year. The first wave hit small

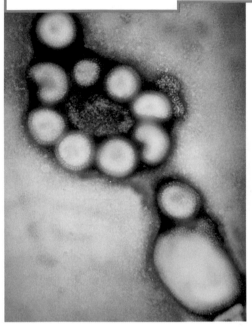

Below, Hong Kong flu viruses are seen at 54,000x magnification. The viruses are surrounded by an envelope of spiked proteins that adhere to host cells during infection.

children, young adults, and pregnant women the hardest. The second wave, which appeared three months later, primarily targeted the elderly. By the time it ended, it had caused approximately seventy thousand deaths in the United States and two million worldwide.

Nearly a decade later, a new flu emerged and spread. In 1968, the A (H3N2) virus first appeared in Hong Kong and, in a matter of months, reached the United States. Deaths peaked over the holiday season, preying mainly on people over the age of sixty-five. By the time the pandemic was brought under control, the Hong Kong flu had caused roughly thirty-four thousand U.S. deaths and one million worldwide.

Near Pandemics

In addition to the certified pandemics discussed above, there have been several other close calls with diseases that threatened to rage out of control. They generated headlines, frightened the public, and placed physicians and hospitals on high alert. Yet they turned out to be far less severe than anticipated, proving that even knowledgeable researchers have difficulty forecasting the extent and progression of a pandemic.

The Swine Flu

In February 1976, soldiers started to get sick at Fort Dix in New Jersey. There were alarming similarities to the outbreak of the Spanish flu, so health officials got scared. They determined that mass inoculation of the public was necessary.

Finding a way to vaccinate 220 million Americans in less than five months was not easy. Since the vaccination for swine flu would have to be made quite rapidly, doctors were unsure what the side effects would be. There was not enough time to conduct the extensive testing that would normally accompany the release of a new vaccine to the public

At the height of the immunization process, their worst fears were realized. Almost a dozen different states began to report an apparent side effect of the swine flu shot—a serious neurological disorder called Guillain-Barre syndrome, which causes temporary progressive ascending muscular weakness (muscle weakness that begins in the extremities—the hands and feet—and can spread to the rest of the body). By the end of 1977, more than 1,098 cases of Guillain-Barre had been diagnosed, resulting in millions of dollars in lawsuits.

The vaccination program was stopped immediately. What had started out as an emergency effort to protect people had turned into an expensive catastrophe. To add insult to injury, the predicted swine flu pandemic never arrived.

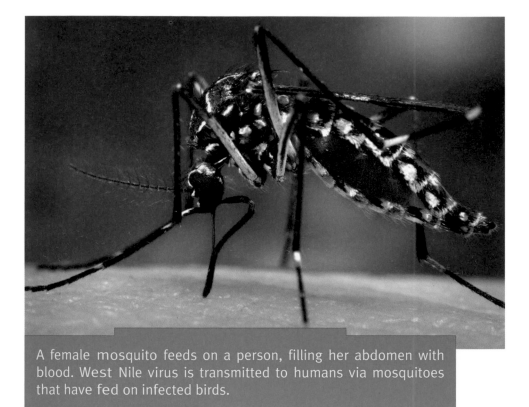

A female mosquito feeds on a person, filling her abdomen with blood. West Nile virus is transmitted to humans via mosquitoes that have fed on infected birds.

West Nile Virus

In 1999, the world had become increasingly uneasy over the threat of the West Nile virus. Carriers of this virus are mosquitoes that have been infected by the birds they landed and fed upon. The West Nile virus is transferred to humans through the bite of infected mosquitoes. Because mosquitoes are only active at certain times of the year, this virus is considered seasonal. There is no treatment for West Nile virus.

Thankfully, the virus has not affected enough people in enough places to qualify as the pandemic some feared it might become. According to the Centers for Disease Control and Prevention (CDC), West Nile's growth and spread has begun to slow. The drop in new cases and fatalities is attributed to anti-mosquito spraying by municipalities and people being aware of the risk of mosquito bites and taking steps to lessen that risk, such as staying indoors at dawn and dusk, wearing long-sleeved shirts and long pants, and spraying themselves and their clothing with insect repellent.

SARS

Beginning in late 2002, hundreds of people in China's Guangdong province began turning up in hospitals with a mysterious respiratory illness. A handful of victims died. In February 2003, a man later referred to by epidemiologists as Patient A traveled from Guangdong province to visit his family in Hong Kong. He infected a dozen people at his hotel. Through their subsequent travels, they in turn spread the illness to Hong Kong, Vietnam, Singapore, Ireland, Germany, and Canada.

Meanwhile, in Hong Kong, ninety-nine cases of this new and very deadly illness appeared, mostly in health care workers. All were connected to a patient who had stayed at the same hotel as Patient A.

This mysterious and deadly condition was eventually named SARS, which stands for sudden acute respiratory syndrome. Researchers determined that SARS was caused by a type of coronavirus, the same family of viruses that causes the common cold.

By mid-March 2003, the World Health Organization (WHO) issued a global SARS alert to travelers who had been in Asia, telling them to watch for possible symptoms. In July, officials

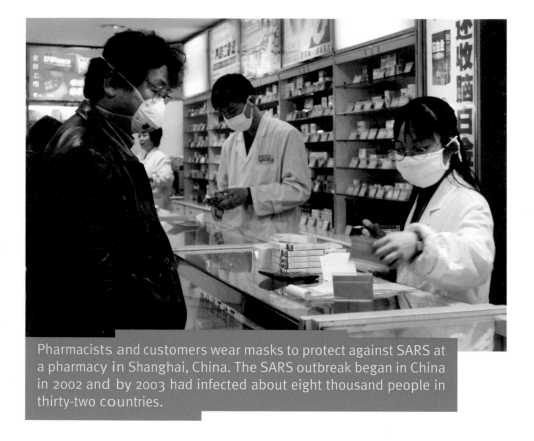

Pharmacists and customers wear masks to protect against SARS at a pharmacy in Shanghai, China. The SARS outbreak began in China in 2002 and by 2003 had infected about eight thousand people in thirty-two countries.

announced that SARS was finally under control. More than eight thousand people had been infected in thirty-two countries, and 744 patients had died.

The SARS outbreak was not extensive or prolonged enough to qualify as an epidemic or a pandemic, but it was sudden and deadly enough to frighten people and get the attention of health organizations around the world. It also severely damaged the Asian economy. Fear over the infectious disease shut down much of the region's daily business and greatly harmed its tourist industry. It is estimated that $30 billion in revenue was lost before the SARS scare was over.

Epidemics and pandemics can be identified, tracked, and studied. However, the one thing they cannot be is predicted with reliability. Sometimes they can look like they are coming straight at us and then miss by a mile. Other times, they really do arrive whether they were anticipated or not.

CHAPTER four

HOW DID AVIAN FLU EMERGE?

The avian flu first appeared in Hong Kong in 1997. Farmers knew something was wrong because their birds were not behaving normally. There was a drop in egg production among the affected birds, and they showed signs of sickness: quietness, swollen or congested combs, swelling of the skin under the eyes, diarrhea, and bleeding. Soon birds began to die in increasing numbers. Then, just as health organizations like the CDC and WHO began to investigate, the virus seemed to fade away. In essence, it dropped out of sight for six years, only to return in 2003. Since December 2003, avian influenza infections in poultry or wild birds have been reported in nearly fifty countries and republics in Africa, East Asia and the Pacific, South Asia, the Near East, Europe, and Eurasia.

Throughout 2004, reports of avian flu cropped up in China and Malaysia. In February 2006, thirteen new

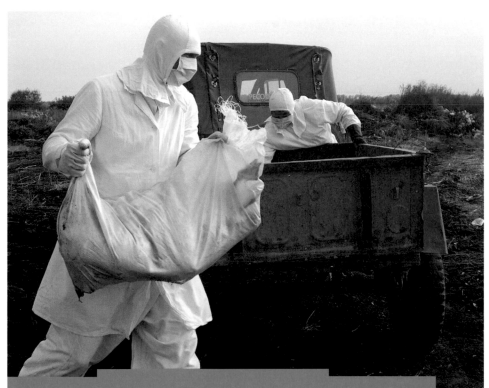

Workers in Russia dispose of dead chickens and ducks infected with avian flu in 2005. Millions of domesticated birds across the world were slaughtered in an attempt to slow the spread of avian flu.

countries reported their first H5N1 infections in wild and domestic birds. Millions of birds have died from either having the virus or being slaughtered because they were suspected of having it. Avian flu has not only killed wild and domesticated birds but also represents a threat to the lives of an untold number of humans.

Bird Flu in Humans

In humans, avian flu symptoms are much like those of any flu, including fever, aches, cough, nasal congestion, sore throat, and respiratory distress. Eye infections and pneumonia may also occur later. With avian flu, the symptoms tend to come on faster and with more intensity than with regular flu. It takes one to five days after exposure to the virus for symptoms to begin appearing.

In May 1997, the first human with avian flu died. Toward the end of 1997, eighteen more people were diagnosed with avian flu, and six of them died. Each patient was shown to have had contact with either a bird's secretions or surfaces where these secretions had been, such as cages, water and feed, or equipment.

A 2006 report issued by the U.S. Department of Health and Human Services stated that the H5N1 virus had been confirmed in 53 countries, with 228 confirmed human cases of avian flu and more than 100 deaths. The most troubling fact in the entire report focused on a flu cluster in an Indonesian family. When a woman contracted the flu following exposure to infected poultry, she infected six other family members. All died but one. Both the WHO and CDC rushed to the scene to administer antivirals to people in the neighboring area and to perform tests to find out how the virus had spread directly from one person to another—a prerequisite for a pandemic. Tests revealed that the virus had mutated slightly in one of the young victims—the first evidence that this was possible. Previous to this, epidemiologists believed that each person who had died of avian flu had some kind of direct contact with diseased birds' saliva, nasal secretions, or feces and that the disease could not yet be transmitted directly from an infected person to a healthy one.

As of 2008, the WHO has reported human cases of avian influenza A in the following countries:

- Cambodia
- China
- Indonesia
- Thailand
- Vietnam
- Azerbaijan
- Turkey
- Egypt
- Iraq
- Djibouti
- Lao People's Democratic Republic
- Myanmar
- Nigeria
- Pakistan

Fortunately, the number of human cases has grown more slowly than that of birds. According to the WHO, as of 2008, 368 people have contracted avian flu, and 234 have died.

The Cost of a Possible Pandemic

As hard as it is to predict whether or not a pandemic is coming, it is even harder to predict what effects it might have if it does arrive. The number of morbidities (incidences of disease) and/or deaths from any pandemic depends on several factors: how many people are infected, how virulent the virus is, how vulnerable a population is, and how effective preventive measures are.

Some researchers and epidemiologists believe it would take about ninety days for a full-fledged avian flu pandemic to sweep across the entire planet, while computer models predict it

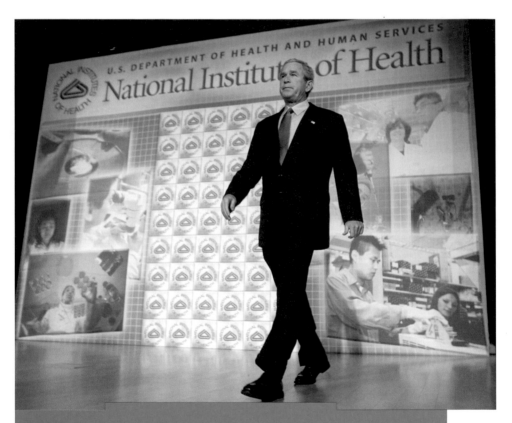

President George W. Bush spoke at the National Institutes of Health in Bethesda, Maryland, in 2005. He encouraged the development of an avian flu vaccine and outlined a strategy to prevent the spread of the disease to the United States.

would be closer to twenty-four days. The CDC and WHO have estimated that if the avian flu should mutate into a human flu, 20 to 47 million humans could become sick, with between 2 million and 7.4 million dying worldwide.

It is also predicted that the cost to the world's economy of a deadly pandemic would range between $71.3 billion and $166.5 billion. Hospitals would be completely overwhelmed, businesses would go bankrupt due to lost workers and customers, and there would probably be significant interruption of such basic services as law enforcement, transportation, communication, and power.

The good news is we are taking steps to be prepared. In October 2005, U.S. president George W. Bush encouraged drug manufacturers to step up the process of creating a bird flu vaccine. The U.S. secretary of health and human services also set up a new service organization called the National Influenza Pandemic Preparedness Task Force. If a bird flu pandemic occurs, we should be in a position to reduce the cost to the world economy and, more important, the number of human lives lost.

HOW HAS AVIAN FLU AFFECTED THE UNITED STATES?

To date, bird flu hasn't been seen anywhere in North America. Even if U.S. chickens were to contract the virus that causes avian flu, there still wouldn't be an automatic pandemic here. In order to catch the disease, a human would have to come into close contact with an infected bird or its feathers and droppings. Also, person-to-person transmission is very rare, even in countries that have seen the virus affect many wild and domesticated birds.

Since the United States has already banned the importing of birds, living or dead, and bird products (such as eggs) from all affected countries, avian flu is not likely to sneak in on grocery shelves. Still, the possibility remains that avian flu could eventually affect birds in North America. Currently, experts believe there are three main ways that the avian flu could get to this country: migratory birds, exotic and illegal bird sales, and cockfighting.

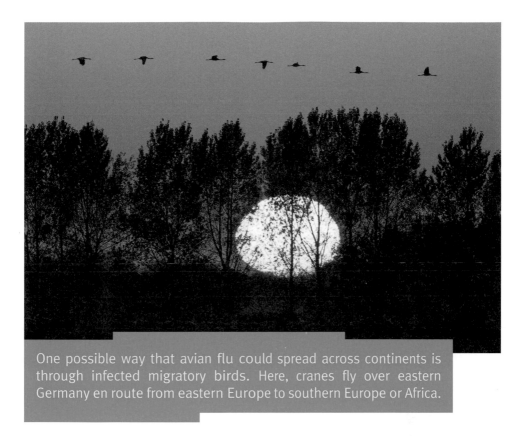

One possible way that avian flu could spread across continents is through infected migratory birds. Here, cranes fly over eastern Germany en route from eastern Europe to southern Europe or Africa.

Migratory Birds

Every autumn, birds fly to regions with warmer climates and then fly back again with the return of spring. This is known as migration. Scientists are worried that migratory birds will pick up the H5N1 virus and spread it wherever they land. The spring migration from Asia to Alaska is particularly worrisome since the flu is so much more prevalent in the Asian regions.

To address this concern, many experts are trying to pinpoint major migratory routes and screen birds as they enter the United

States. Although they are currently examining five to six times as many birds as they did just a few years ago, it is still an overwhelming project. In addition, migratory routes cannot always be predicted. They can vary from year to year and can be quite complex.

Sales of Exotic Birds

Statistics show that 400,000 live exotic birds are imported to the United States each year as pets. At least a quarter of these birds come in illegally. According to the government, wildlife smuggling ranks in profitability second only to illegal drug trafficking.

United States regulations require that all imported wild birds must spend thirty days in government quarantine stations to make sure they are healthy. Obviously, with birds smuggled in secretly and illegally, there is no opportunity for such quarantine and protection. If someone smuggles in birds that carry the H5N1 virus, the infections could quickly spread to other birds in this country. This, in turn, would increase the chance of the virus mutating enough to be able to infect humans.

Cockfighting

The third way that avian flu could spread quickly in the United States is through cockfighting, in which two roosters are placed in a ring so they will fight each other. People place bets on which rooster will win.

Cockfighting is hugely popular throughout Asia, particularly in Thailand and the Philippines. Although cockfighting is illegal in forty-eight states, it is still legal in Louisiana and New Mexico. It is performed illegally in many more states as well. Each day,

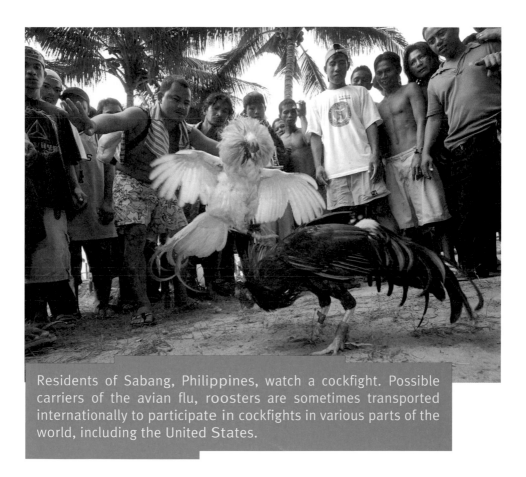

Residents of Sabang, Philippines, watch a cockfight. Possible carriers of the avian flu, roosters are sometimes transported internationally to participate in cockfights in various parts of the world, including the United States.

tens of thousands of fighting birds travel across the country. If they happen to be infected, H5N1 would go along for the ride, too. Since fighting cocks can earn their owners a lot of money, they are often well cared for and frequently handled. If a bird is injured, the handler will often come into direct contact with the rooster's blood, which can transmit the avian flu virus.

It is likely that with these three areas of national vulnerability—migration, illegal imports, and cockfighting—bird flu will reach the United States sooner rather than later. Will the country be ready? No one is quite sure.

Myths and Facts

 Myth **All migratory birds carry avian influenza.**
Fact ➡ The role of migratory birds in the spread of avian flu is still unclear. It is true that wild waterfowl are considered to be the natural carriers of all influenza A viruses. They are known to carry the subtypes H5 and H7. However, these are usually in a low pathogenic (mild) form. While some migratory birds may be spreading the influenza H5N1 virus, it is doubtful that all of them are.

 Myth **Poultry products can transfer the flu to humans.**
Fact ➡ Influenza viruses cannot be passed through properly cooked food. Even if the food was contaminated, the virus cannot survive the heat from the cooking process.

 Myth **It's easy for humans to become infected with avian flu.**
Fact ➡ It is not easy for humans to become infected with avian flu. Even people who have

handled infected birds often do not become infected themselves.

Some of the best information about the avian flu is on the Internet. Fact ●→ This could be true, depending on where you do your surfing. Government and public health sites like the Centers for Disease Control and Prevention, the World Health Organization, and the newly created www.pandemicflu.gov, or news sites like CNN or BBC give reliable reports and updates. Unfortunately, there are also a lot of Web sites that are full of sensationalistic rumors, misleading statements, and exaggerated statistics. For instance, companies claim they've created cures for the coming bird flu, or e-books declare that for $4.95 you can find the one surefire way to prevent ever getting sick. Such wild claims often lead to even wilder fears.

Current flu vaccines will protect people from the avian flu. Fact ●→ Modern flu vaccines are designed to provide some protection against seasonal flu strains. However, they have nothing in them that would help anyone stay safe from the bird flu. A vaccine specifically made to counteract the bird flu has not yet been produced, though research and development are well underway.

Feathers are safe to be touched and handled.
Fact ➡ Because a bird's secretions can get on its feathers, they are actually considered risky to handle. If you do not know where feathers came from, avoid touching them.

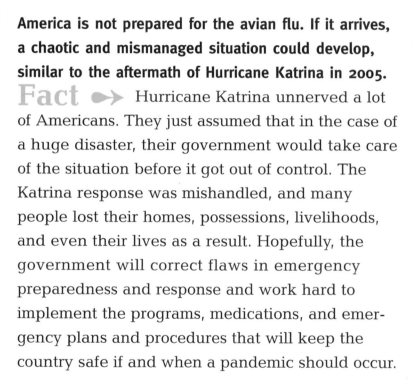

America is not prepared for the avian flu. If it arrives, a chaotic and mismanaged situation could develop, similar to the aftermath of Hurricane Katrina in 2005.
Fact ➡ Hurricane Katrina unnerved a lot of Americans. They just assumed that in the case of a huge disaster, their government would take care of the situation before it got out of control. The Katrina response was mishandled, and many people lost their homes, possessions, livelihoods, and even their lives as a result. Hopefully, the government will correct flaws in emergency preparedness and response and work hard to implement the programs, medications, and emergency plans and procedures that will keep the country safe if and when a pandemic should occur.

The avian flu will be as devastating as the 1918 Spanish flu. Fact ➡ Fortunately, this is not true. Although there are definite similarities, there are also very important differences that make the avian flu much less of a threat. The medical, informational, technological, and emergency response resources of the twenty-first-century world are vastly superior to those available in 1918.

CHAPTER SIX

WHAT ARE SOME STRATEGIES AND TREATMENTS?

Although media reports and talk on the street may make it sound like people are powerless in the battle against an avian flu pandemic, that is just not true. With each passing day, it becomes even less true. There are a number of ways that we can protect against the devastation of an avian flu pandemic. Most of these measures—such as culling any birds that have been exposed to H5N1 or show symptoms of the flu—have been in place for more than a year in many affected countries.

Close surveillance systems have also been set up. An international surveillance system currently exists in more than 150 countries. The United States has launched the National Bio-Surveillance Initiative. The people who work in this system have been trained to watch for three distinct things: multiple cases of a single illness, more severe illnesses than usual, and incidents of flu that occur outside the typical winter season.

Containment

One of the best ways to avoid a pandemic or to reduce its extent is containment. This is when plans are put into action that help prevent the virus from spreading. These include keeping infected people away from those who are healthy in what's known as isolation or quarantine.

In addition to quarantines, governments and other decision makers may try social distancing, which is halting normal activities where many people gather together and might pass on the virus through social contact. This could mean closing schools and offices, canceling sporting events, closing movie theaters, and shutting down mass transportation. There would also likely be tougher restrictions placed on immigration and international travel. Those who were traveling from countries strongly affected by the pandemic could possibly be denied entry into the country, and those who arrived looking ill might be placed in quarantine.

Tracing where an infected person has been within the past few weeks is also part of containment. People who live near or have had direct contact with someone who has avian flu would be given prophylactic (preventative) antiviral drugs because they would be at an increased risk of getting the virus. In fact, people within large areas of where virus infections have occurred would be given shots in an attempt to keep more people from getting the flu.

Containment methods for the avian flu virus, should it appear, include quarantining or isolating infected communities, as well as travel restrictions, school and airport closures, limited public gatherings, and curfews. Trying to contain an emerging pandemic virus takes a lot of work, not to mention patience and time. Decision makers have to be absolutely sure that conditions are right for a pandemic before putting drastic and disruptive containment measures into effect.

A Future Vaccine

Vaccines are being developed and stockpiled. In August 2005, the U.S. government agreed to purchase millions of doses of a prototype bird flu vaccine created and sold by a French manufacturer. It is a very potent vaccine—more than six times the strength of typical vaccines—and is based on a current strain of the avian flu. If and when the drug is approved for sale and human use, it will take another six to twelve months to get it into production.

No one is sure how effective an avian flu vaccine would be. Until then, they can only guess at how the virus may mutate to make person-to-person contact possible and how those mutations may alter the strength and progression of the illness.

Antiviral Medications

One way flu has been mitigated (made less severe) in the past is through antiviral medications such as amantadine, rimantadine, oseltamivir (Tamiflu), and zanamivir (Relenza). Each one has both benefits and negative side effects. Although none of them

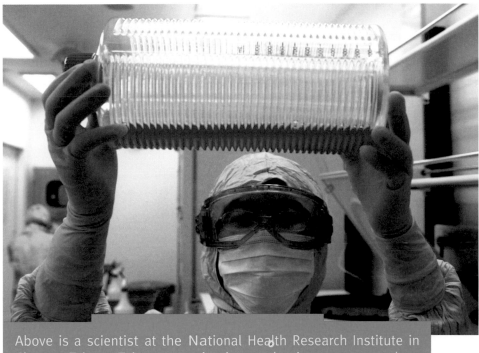

Above is a scientist at the National Health Research Institute in Chunan, Taiwan. Taiwanese scientists are hoping to mass-produce a bird flu vaccine in the near future.

can prevent people from getting the flu, they can lessen the severity and duration of the symptoms.

Amantadine has been on the market since 1976. It interferes with a virus's ability to replicate, or make copies of itself. It has been reported to cause nervousness, anxiety, insomnia, and light-headedness. Rimantadine, which came on the market in 1993, works the same way as amantadine. Unfortunately, about 12 percent of people are resistant to this medication.

Tamiflu is an antiviral drug that can lessen the severity of avian flu symptoms.

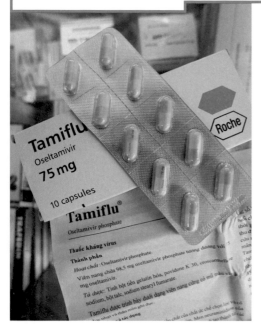

Both Tamiflu and Relenza were released in 1999, and they work to block the enzyme that the virus needs in order to escape from one cell and infect another. Relenza is an inhaled powder, which makes it hard to administer to people who are already coughing and having trouble breathing.

Tamiflu seems to be the most effective antiviral drug, and it is the one the government is stockpiling. Currently, the WHO has between three and five million doses of it for use at the first sign of an avian flu outbreak.

Immune System

The immune system is your body's defense system against disease. When it is working properly, it finds and fights pathogenic, or disease-causing, organisms such as bacteria, viruses, parasites, and fungi. Your immune system gives you the strength, energy, and power to fight minor illnesses such as colds. A

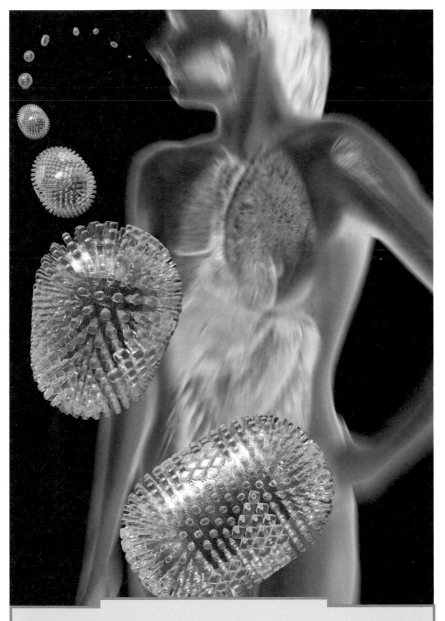

In this diagram of an avian flu infection, airborne viruses *(green)* enter the lungs *(olive green)*, causing a huge influx of immune proteins called cytokines into the lung tissue.

healthy immune system can also detect and repair damaged cells, such as ones that have been injured by cancer and other diseases.

Serious problems can occur when your immune system is weakened. You may experience frequent or long-lasting infections—ones that recur over months or won't go away at all. A compromised immune system may fail to detect the growth of unhealthy cells, resulting in cancer. The body's immune system cannot fight off cancer, so therapies, such as chemotherapy or radiation therapy, are then used to complete the job of fighting disease.

Your immune system is your body's way of defending your health and keeping you alive, so it's important to understand how it works. It is a very complicated network of organs and cells that work together to fight deadly intruders called antigens, which are any foreign thing that could make you sick, like bacteria, fungi, parasites, or viruses. Once inside the cells of a host, a virus tries to become active and multiply. If it is successful, it can eventually create so many copies of itself that it causes the cell to burst, releasing the virus into the body. Then the virus finds more cells in your body in which to live. This process can continue until the virus has attacked enough cells to make you ill. However, a healthy and strong immune system can usually kill any viruses before they multiply to such a damaging degree.

Natural Antivirals

If you want to start on your own immune boosters, you don't have to wait for your physician to give you a prescription. There are some supplements that you can get at your local health food store and use on a daily basis:

Many studies have shown that green tea can help boost your immune system.

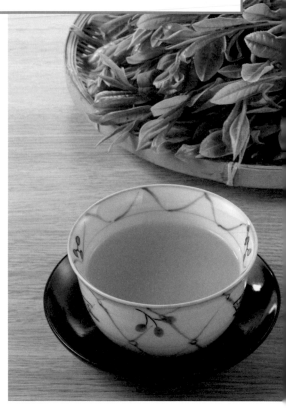

- Garlic (raw)
- Vitamin C
- Green tea
- Saint-John's-wort
- Apple juice
- Skullcap

These natural substances help boost your immune system. They won't protect you against the avian flu virus, but they may increase your general health and strengthen your immune system, possibly making you less vulnerable to infection.

Feeling helpless in the face of a potential pandemic may be understandable, but it is also mistaken. Hundreds of people are putting plans into place, from doctors and nurses at the local clinic down the street to the heads of the federal government in Washington, D.C. Keep informed and keep calm. Information and help will be there when—or if—you need them.

Ten Great Questions to Ask Your Doctor

1 How is avian flu transmitted to humans?

2 When do you think an avian flu vaccine will be available to the general public?

3 What do you think is the most effective method for treating avian flu in people?

4 Does your office currently have a plan in place for patients should this pandemic occur?

5 What precautions should I be taking right now to help lessen the risk of the bird flu?

6 What books relating to the bird flu would you recommend?

7 Are there any alternative treatments you can suggest that might boost my immune system?

8 How effective do you think the government's pandemic plan is?

9 Would a quarantine be helpful in our community?

10 What plans have you personally made in preparation for a possible pandemic?

seven

HOW CAN I STAY SAFE AND CALM?

Are you worried about the avian flu now? Do the evening news reports and newspaper and magazine articles make you feel like doom may be just around the corner? Do you comb online news sites for new information that indicates a pandemic is imminent? If so, you may be making yourself unwell even without coming into contact with the flu virus.

An Epidemic of Fear

Although the dangers of catching avian flu in North America are real, they are also, at this point, extremely unlikely. The avian flu may arrive in the United States, and it may not. If it does arrive, it may make the leap from birds to humans, or it may not.

Being terribly worried and constantly afraid, however, is a real and immediate danger. It can cause emotional and physical stress, resulting in high blood pressure, chest pain, anxiety, shortness of breath, headache, and even depression. Dr. Marc Siegel wrote in his book *Bird Flu: Everything You Need to Know About the Next Pandemic*, "The greatest problem among my patients right now isn't bird flu; it is fear of bird flu. The greatest risk of an epidemic is a fear epidemic . . . Fear is infectious." He continued, "Fear of bird flu has become particularly virulent. There is a vaccine for this fear: it is called information mixed with perspective. Since there is a shortage of this vaccine, fear has begun to spread throughout my community and yours. That is a chilling foretaste of the horror of a true epidemic."

While burying your head in the sand or ignoring what is going on is not the wisest course, neither is obsessing about the possibility of a pandemic. As Dr. Anthony Fauci, director of the National Institute of Allergy and Infectious Diseases at the National Institutes of Health, stated to *USA Today*, "The one thing I can say is that you often hear that we're one mutation away from having a pandemic that spreads everywhere. Well, yes and no. Let me concentrate on the no. That implies that it's a very simple event to get a virus that is very poorly transmissible to become highly transmissible. No, a lot of different things have to happen to that virus for it to be able to go from very poorly efficient to highly efficient." Continued Fauci, "Health officials like myself have to assume a) That will happen and b) It will be a worst-case scenario because you have to gear up your preparation. But when the American public gets up in the morning and goes to work, they should not be fixating that we're one mutation away from disaster."

The three typical ways that the public reacts to a disaster like a pandemic are:

1. **Denial:** "There's no way this is really happening. It is just being overhyped by the media."
2. **Hysteria:** "This will be just like Hurricane Katrina. We are doomed. No one will help us."
3. **Optimism, rationality, and pragmatism:** "I need to hope for the best and prepare for the worst!"

The third reaction is the healthiest and most prudent. It is important to balance legitimate cause for concern with equally legitimate reasons for confidence and optimism. A close examination of the many differences that exist between the 1918 Spanish flu disaster and today's threat of avian flu highlights both the areas of greater concern and those that offer reassurance that a large-scale, worldwide catastrophe is unlikely.

Reasons for Optimism and Confidence

Happily, the world has changed dramatically since 1918, when the Spanish flu ravaged the world. We have at our disposal many more resources that greatly facilitate doing battle with worldwide pandemics. Consider the following positive factors:

The Internet allows for the dissemination of immediate, worldwide information and instructions on quarantine locations, clinics offering immunization, how to avoid

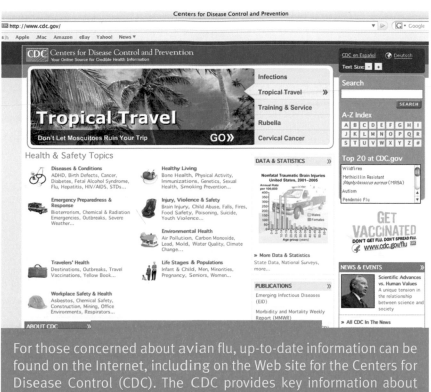

For those concerned about avian flu, up-to-date information can be found on the Internet, including on the Web site for the Centers for Disease Control (CDC). The CDC provides key information about many infectious diseases.

crowds, and other vital facts that will assist in limiting the effects and spread of an epidemic.

➤ Sanitation and hygiene have greatly improved in most parts of the world since 1918.

➤ Doctors are more knowledgeable about the nature of viruses and disease, infection and epidemics, and the treatment required to fight specific illnesses.

➤ Experts have gathered and analyzed important data from previous pandemics and learned valuable lessons as a result.

➤ Hospitals already have pandemic emergency plans in place, which will be activated the moment signs of a local outbreak become apparent.

➤ Countries all over the world are monitoring the situation and are sharing information.

➤ Antiviral drugs exist and are being manufactured and stock-piled for potential use.

Being Prepared

Avian flu and the threat of a pandemic can make you feel paralyzed by anxiety and uncertainty. One of the best ways to combat this worry is to feel more in control and do something active to address the issue. Reading reliable and up-to-date information from good sources is essential. Learning as much as we can about the realities (and the rumors) surrounding this flu is the best way for us to respond.

While there is no vaccine to line up for yet, you can still take some concrete steps to begin fighting avian flu. For example, you can have an emergency plan ready should the pandemic begin and affect your local area. You can ask your physician questions and discuss your thoughts, fears, and action plan with your parents, teachers, or friends. The American Red Cross is one of the best resources for learning how to put together an emergency preparedness kit. Here are the basics of what you should keep on hand in order to weather an avian flu pandemic (should one arrive) and the resulting disruptions to your community and your daily routine:

A first-aid kit is handy to have around for everyday situations and could also prove useful in the event of an avian flu outbreak.

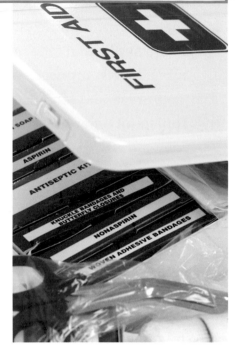

Water: You will need water for keeping clean, preparing food, and staying hydrated. A good guideline to follow is one gallon of water per day per adult. Don't forget that you will need more if you have pets.

Food: While you can go several weeks without eating (as opposed to only a few days without water), you will be better and more comfortably able to weather any prolonged confinement to your house or restricted opportunities to get fresh provisions if you have some supplies on hand. Experts recommend a three-day supply of nonperishable foods (requiring no refrigeration, cooking, or preparation to eat). Suggestions include canned juices, fruits, and vegetables, and high-energy foods such as granola bars and peanut butter. Remember a nonelectric can opener, too.

First-aid supplies: It's a good rule to have a first-aid kit on hand for any kind of common household emergency such as cuts, scrapes, splinters, pulled muscles, sprained ankles, etc.—not just something as relatively unlikely as the avian flu. It should include bandages, sterile dressings, gauze pads, antibacterial wet wipes, antibacterial ointment, non-latex gloves, tape, scissors, tweezers, thermometer, aspirin, cough syrup, and face masks. Other things to remember are contact lens supplies, an extra pair of eyeglasses, and a toothbrush and toothpaste.

Tools and emergency supplies: Set aside a storage area in your house—perhaps the basement or pantry—to stow items such as disposable cups, plates, and utensils, along with a battery-operated radio, a flashlight, cash, various types of batteries, a tool kit, a fire extinguisher, matches, toilet paper, soap, detergent, and disinfectant for emergency use. These supplies also come in handy in the event of other emergencies, like hurricanes, tornadoes, or snowstorms.

Paperwork: In an emergency—and especially if you have to evacuate your house—you family may need quick access to important documents, such as wills, insurance policies, deeds, stocks and bonds, medical records and information, passports, Social Security cards, identification cards, tax returns, banking account numbers, credit card account numbers, important phone numbers, and birth, marriage, and death certificates. Have copies of these materials stored in a file folder and placed in a location you can easily remember and access.

Pets: Be sure to store at least several days' worth of food, water, medication, and plastic bags (for waste) needed by your pets. Collect and file their veterinary records.

➥ **Entertainment:** Time will seem to crawl if you are quarantined or isolated and have not made any provision for distracting yourself. Pack nonelectronic forms of entertainment such as books, games, a deck of cards, plenty of paper, and several pens. You probably won't want to waste precious and limited battery power on video games or music.

It is always wise, in every circumstance, to follow the Boy Scout motto: Be prepared. It is much better to have something on hand and not need it than to need it and not have it.

Other Tips for Staying Safe and Healthy

Keep in mind at all times that at this point the danger avian flu poses to Americans is minimal. It has not yet been reported in the United States. Even in the most affected countries, the number of infections and deaths is not large. There are many people working hard to develop an effective vaccine. And in the unlikely event that you do become infected with the avian flu virus, there are several medications that your doctor can give you.

One of the best things you can do to lessen your risk of getting the bird flu—or any flu, for that matter—is to stay healthy. You can do this through getting enough sleep, eating the healthiest diet possible, and avoiding harmful substances like tobacco, alcohol, and drugs.

Other suggestions for staying safe include regularly disinfecting surfaces of your house (such as countertops, cutting boards, sinks,

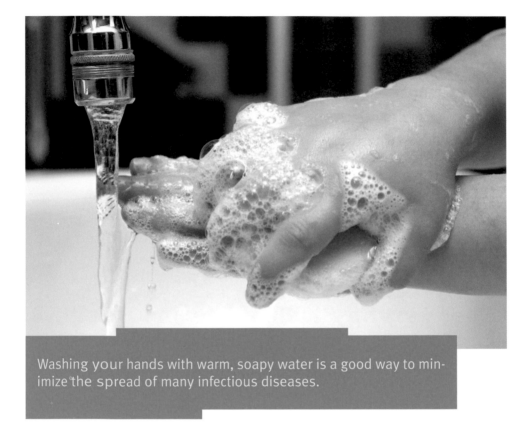

Washing your hands with warm, soapy water is a good way to minimize the spread of many infectious diseases.

and toilets) to lessen the potential germs there. Wash your hands several times a day with soap. Be sure to cough and sneeze into a tissue, and stay at home if you are sick.

Remember that fear is the biggest obstacle to staying healthy. As Dr. Marc Siegel wrote in *Avian Flu: Everything You Need to Know About the Next Pandemic*, "The fear surrounding avian flu comes not from what is currently happening, but from what-if scenarios." Live your life, enjoy each day to its fullest, prepare for what events seem likely to come to pass, and don't worry about what you can't control or foresee. You can trust yourself to be able to deal with whatever comes your way, especially if you've already prepared for the most likely occurrences. Until it is time to deal with a problem, enjoy your life, have fun with your family and friends, and stay happy and healthy. You'll be far better prepared to deal with challenges if you have this positive and pragmatic outlook on life.

Glossary

antigenic drift Small, permanent, ongoing changes in the genetic material of a virus strain that are considered normal.

antigenic shift Sudden, major changes in a virus's genetic makeup; this is often the cause in flu epidemics.

antiviral Destroying or inhibiting the growth and reproduction of viruses.

domesticated Describes an animal that has learned how to live in a human environment.

epidemic Spreading rapidly and extensively by infection and affecting many individuals in an area or a population at the same time.

inoculate To introduce a serum, vaccine, or antigenic substance into the body of a person or animal to produce or boost immunity to a specific disease.

mutate To change.

outbreak A sudden increase in incidence of a disease.

pandemic Epidemic over a wide area, usually global.

pathogen An agent that causes disease such as a bacterium, fungus, parasite, or virus.

quarantine A period of time during which a vehicle, person, animal, or material suspected of carrying a contagious disease is detained at a port of entry under enforced isolation to prevent disease from entering a country.

SARS Acronym for sudden acute respiratory syndrome.

stockpile A supply stored for future use, usually carefully gathered and maintained.

surveillance Close observation of a person, group, or situation.

susceptible Likely to be affected; especially sensitive.

vaccine A substance made from a weakened or dead virus or bacterium that makes the body produce more antibodies, which fight disease and infection.

virulent Extremely infectious, malignant, or poisonous.

virus A small pathogen composed of protein and nucleic acid that lives off of other organisms, reproduces very quickly, and causes disease.

Centers for Disease Control and Prevention
1600 Clifton Road
Atlanta, GA 30333
(800) 311-3435
Web site: http://www.cdc.gov

The Centers for Disease Control and Prevention (CDC) is at
the forefront of public health efforts to prevent and control
infectious and chronic diseases, injuries, workplace hazards,
disabilities, and environmental health threats.

National Institute of Allergy and Infectious Diseases
National Institutes of Health
Office of Communications and Public Liaison
6610 Rockledge Drive, MSC 6612
Bethesda, MD 20892-6612
(301) 496-5717
Web site: http://www3.niaid.nih.gov

The National Institute of Allergy and Infectious Diseases
(NIAID) conducts and supports research to better understand, treat, and ultimately prevent infectious, immunologic,
and allergic diseases. NIAID research has led to new
therapies, vaccines, diagnostic tests, and other technologies
that have improved the health of millions of people in the
United States and around the world.

U.S. Department of Agriculture
1400 Independence Avenue SW
Washington, DC 20205
Web site: http://www.usda.gov/wps/portal/usdahome
   The Department of Agriculture provides leadership on food,
   agriculture, natural resources, and related issues based on
   sound public policy, the best available science, and efficient
   management. Among other things, it seeks to enhance food
   safety by taking steps to reduce the prevalence of foodborne
   hazards from farm to table.

U.S. Department of Health and Human Services
200 Independence Avenue SW
Washington, DC 20201
(877) 696-6775
Web site: http://www.hhs.gov
   The Department of Health and Human Services is the U.S.
   government's principal agency for protecting the health of all
   Americans and providing essential human services.

U.S. Geological Survey National Wildlife Health Center
6006 Schroeder Road
Madison, WI 53711-6223
(608) 270-2400
Web site: http://www.nwhc.usgs.gov
   The U.S. Geological Survey serves the nation by providing
   reliable scientific information to describe and understand Earth;
   minimize loss of life and property from natural disasters;

manage water, biological, energy, and mineral resources; and enhance and protect our quality of life.

World Health Organization
Regional Office for the Americas
525 23rd Street NW
Washington, DC 20037
(202) 974-3000
Web site: http://www.who.int/en/
   The World Health Organization is the United Nations' specialized agency for health. Its objective is the attainment by all peoples of the highest possible level of health, defined by the organization as a state of complete physical, mental, and social well-being and not merely the absence of disease or infirmity.

Web Sites

Due to the changing nature of Internet links, Rosen Publishing has developed an online list of Web sites related to the subject of this book. This site is updated regularly. Please use this link to access the list:

http://www.rosenlinks.com/faq/avfl

For Further Reading

Altshuler, Laurence H. *The Bird-Flu Primer: The Guide to Being Prepared and Surviving an Avian Flu Epidemic.* New York, NY: Sterling and Ross Publications, 2006.

Barry, John M. *The Great Influenza: The Epic Story of the Deadliest Plague in History.* New York, NY: Viking, 2004.

Boire, Martin C. *How to Survive the Bird Flu.* Daytona Beach, FL: MemoMania, LLC, 2005.

Crosby, Alfred W. *America's Forgotten Pandemic: The Influenza of 1918.* New York, NY: Cambridge University Press, 2003.

Davis, Mike. *The Monster at Our Door: The Global Threat of Avian Flu.* New York, NY: New Press, 2005.

Sfakinos, Jeffrey N. *Avian Flu.* New York, NY: Chelsea House Publications, 2006.

Siegel, Marc, M.D. *Bird Flu: Everything You Need to Know About the Next Pandemic.* Hoboken, NJ: John Wiley and Sons, 2006.

Silverstein, Alan. *The Flu and Pneumonia Update.* Berkeley Heights, NJ: Enslow Publishers, 2006.

Woodson, Grattan, M.D. *The Bird Flu Preparedness Planner.* Deerfield Beach, FL: HCI, 2005.

Index

Photo Credits